CONTENTS

DRINK TEA.

HIBISCUS TEA

EAT MORE BEETS.

DASH DIET

GRAINS; 6 TO 8 SERVINGS A DAY

VEGETABLES: 4 TO 5 SERVINGS A DAY

NATURAL PRODUCTS: 4 TO 5 SERVINGS A DAY

DAIRY: 2 TO 3 SERVINGS A DAY

INCLINE MEAT, POULTRY AND FISH: 6 OR LESS SERVINGS A DAY

PHYSICAL ACTION TO LOWER BLOOD PRESSURE AND SHED POUNDS

GO FOR POWER STROLLS

BLOOD PRESSURE, BREATHING, AND ANXIETY ADMINISTRATION

LITTLE CHANGES AND ACTIVITIES TO ADOPT TO BRING DOWN YOUR BLOOD PRESSURE

BE SALT KEEN

ENJOY DIM CHOCOLATE

DRINK (A BIT) LIQUOR

WORK (SOMEWHAT) LESS

UNWIND WITH MUSIC

LOOK FOR HELP FOR WHEEZING

BOUNCE FOR SOY

CONCLUSION

Book Description

Agonized over your steadily expanding Blood Pressure? Searching for approaches to lower and keep up your blood pressure? Nourished up of relying upon prescriptions to enhance your wellbeing? Worried about contracting cardio vascular illnesses or diabetes on account of hypertension? Not certain how to lessen your anxiety levels and body weight keeping in mind the end goal to bring down your blood pressure? This book is your definitive arrangement and the response to every one of your questions.

Of the incalculable diseases that rack the human machine, hypertension is one of the least demanding to avoid and a standout amongst the most receptive to treatment. Who gets hypertension? Should you freeze in the event that you or somebody you cherish creates hypertension? In what manner would you be able to help yourself, regardless of the possibility that you're in a high-hazard bunch? This book will answer every one of your inquiries.

Hypertension is ordinarily the aftereffect of an undesirable way of life, and it can quite often be controlled- - without incapacitating medicines - just by eating the right nourishments, taking the best possible herb and vitamin supplements, getting the right sorts of activity, and rehearsing such push lessening methods presently, kendo, and yoga. This book gives you a firm grasp on every one of these instruments. Begin utilizing them today to construct you a solid, dissemination amicable life.

This is the thing that you will learn in this book:

- What is Blood Pressure?

- Who is at a danger of growing high BP?

- What are the symptoms of hypertension?

- What are the advantages of bringing down high BP?

- How to utilize a Blood Pressure Screen at home?

- What's the best eating routine arrangement to take after for hypertension

- How physical action is a key element to returning to a sheltered blood pressure

- How weight administration can help with hypertension

- How decreasing your anxiety levels can be a key element to diminishing hypertension

- 15 super nourishments that can help diminish hypertension

INTRODUCTION

Meds are not by any means the only answer for treating all wellbeing conditions. Individuals have customarily utilized numerous home grown cures and other common answers for battle maladies and lead a sound way of life. Hypertension or hypertension, particularly, is a wellbeing condition for which even specialists prescribe exchange treatments notwithstanding the drugs they recommend. Getting into an activity administration, rehearsing anxiety help methods, embracing a sound eating regimen like the Dash eating regimen, taking home grown supplements, exchanging your cooking oil, stopping smoking, frequently observing your BP at home and so on are certain shot approaches to diminish hoisted blood pressure in your body. Regardless of the possibility that you are under solution, it is recommended that you incorporate normal and solid treatments to decrease your hypertension. This book would take you through the essentials of Blood Pressure.

We should simply be genuine for a second…if you have hypertension, it can be frightening now and again, and particularly when your specialist lets you know that you are currently at a high hazard for a heart assault. Granted, specialists can recommend pills to help briefly, yet pills don't get to the base of the issue. The most ideal approach to bring down your blood pressure is through regular systems, and we can offer assistance!

This book is a regulated book that will take you by the hand and demonstrate to you precisely industry standards to take control of your blood pressure so you don't need to live in apprehension any more. The issue with most books on this theme is they toss a considerable measure of data at you yet they never give you a reasonable activity arrangement. When you are done perusing this book on actually bringing down your blood pressure, you will know precisely what you have to do beginning today to bring down your blood pressure and carry on with a long and cheerful life.

None of the things in this book are troublesome; they simply include rolling out some way of life improvements. These progressions are anything but difficult to make and keep up for the long haul, which is the thing that you will need to do to keep up your blood pressure at a more typical level. There are likewise some convenient formulas at the back of this book which are all intended to be low in fat and sodium to be suitable for individuals why should attempting decrease their blood pressure.

Chapter 1: Blood Pressure – The Basics

What is Blood Pressure?

Blood is conveyed from the heart to all parts of your body in vessels called courses. Blood pressure is the power of the blood pushing against the dividers of the arteries. Every time the heart thumps (around 60-70 times each moment very still), it pumps out blood into the conduits. Your blood pressure is grinding away most astoundingly when the heart pulsates, pumping the blood. This is called systolic pressure. At the point when the heart is very still, between thumps, your blood pressure falls. This is the diastolic pressure.

Blood pressure is constantly given presently numbers, the systolic and diastolic pressures. Both are critical. Normally they are composed one above or before the other, for example, 120/80 mmHg. The top number is the systolic and the base the diastolic. At the point when the two estimations are composed down the systolic pressure is the first and the diastolic pressure is the second or base number (for instance, 120/80). In the event that your blood pressure is 120/80, you say that it is "120 more than 80."

Blood pressure changes amid the day. It is least presently and rises when you get up. It additionally can rise when you are energized, apprehensive, or dynamic.

Still, for the greater part of your waking hours, your blood pressure stays basically the same when you are sitting or stopping and that level ought to be lower than 120/80. At the point when the level stays high 140/90 or higher, it means you have hypertension. With hypertension, the heart lives up to expectations harder, your conduits get destroyed, and your possibilities of a stroke, heart assault, and kidney issues are more prominent.

Causes of Hypertension

In numerous individuals with hypertension, a solitary particular reason is not known. This is called fundamental or essential hypertension. Exploration is keeping on discovering reasons.

In a few individuals, hypertension is the aftereffect of another therapeutic issue or medicine. At the point when the reason is known, this is called auxiliary hypertension.

Hypertension, likewise called hypertension, is unsafe on the grounds that it makes the heart work harder to pump blood out to the body and adds to solidifying of the conduits, or atherosclerosis, to stroke, kidney infection, and to the advancement of heart failure.

The accurate reasons for hypertension are not known, but rather a few variables and conditions may assume a part in its improvement, including:

- Smoking
- Being overweight or large
- Absence of physical movement
- An excessive amount of salt in the eating regimen
- An excessive amount of liquor utilization (more than 1 to 2 beverages fc every day)
- Stress
- More seasoned age
- Hereditary qualities
- Family history of hypertension
- Incessant kidney illness
- Adrenal and thyroid issue
- Rest apnea
- Key Hypertension

These dangers and risk factors are explained in detail below:

FAMILY HISTORY

Tallness, hair and eye shading runs in families and so can hypertension. On the off chance that your folks or close blood relatives have had HBP, you are more inclined to create it, as well. You may additionally pass that hazard consider on to your kids. That is the reason it's imperative for youngsters and grown-ups to have general blood pressure checks. You can't control heredity, however you can make moves to carry on with a solid life and bring down your other danger elements.

Way of life-decisions has permitted numerous individuals with an in number family history of HBP to maintain a strategic distance from it themselves. Find out about way of life changes you can make to avoid HBP. Eye shading isn't your just acquired quality. You might likewise share a danger for HBP.

PROPELLED AGE

Right now, we all create higher danger for hypertension and cardiovascular sickness. Blood vessels lose adaptability with age which can add to expanding pressure all through the framework.

A higher rate of men than ladies have HBP until 45 years old. From ages 45 to 54 and 55 to 64, the rates of men and ladies with HBP are comparative. After that, a much higher rate of ladies have HBP than men.

ABSENCE OF PHYSICAL MOVEMENT

Physical movement is useful for your heart and circulatory framework. An inert way of life expands the possibility of hypertension, coronary illness, blood vessel infection and stroke. Latency additionally makes it simpler to end up overweight or stout. Give yourself the endowment of enhanced wellbeing and lower blood pressure with consistent, moderate-to-enthusiastic physical action.

To nurture our bodies, we all need great nourishment from an assortment of sustenance sources. An eating routine that is high in calories, fats and sugars and low in crucial supplements contributes straightforwardly to weakness and in addition to corpulence. What's more, there are a few issues that can happen from eating a lot of salt. A few individuals are "salt touchy," significance a high-salt (sodium) eating routine raises their hypertension. Salt keeps abundance liquid in the body that can include to the weight the heart. While an excess of salt can be hazardous, sound sustenance decisions can really lower blood pressure. Find out about getting a charge out of a heart-sound eating routine.

An eating routine high in sodium and low in wholesome quality puts you at higher danger for HBP.

OVERWEIGHT AND STOUTNESS

Being overweight expands your shots of growing hypertension. A body mass file somewhere around 25 and 30 is viewed as overweight. A body mass record more than 30 is viewed as stout. Around 66% of U.S. grown-ups are overweight or stout. Around one in three U.S. kids ages 2 to 19 are overweight or stout. Abundance weight expands the strain on the heart, raises blood cholesterol and triglyceride levels, and brings down HDL (great) cholesterol levels. It can likewise make diabetes more prone to create. Losing as meager at this very moment 20 pounds can help bring down your blood pressure and your coronary illness hazard. To effectively and invigoratingly get more fit—and keep it off—a great many people need to subtract around 500 calories for every day from their eating routine to lose around 1 pound for each week. Ascertain your body mass record and figure out how to deal with your weight.

DRINKING AN EXCESSIVE AMOUNT OF LIQUOR

Substantial and general utilization of liquor can build blood pressure drastically. It can likewise bring about heart failure, lead to stroke and produce unpredictable heartbeats. A lot of liquor can add to high triglycerides, disease and different illnesses, weight, liquor abuse, suicide and mischance. On the off chance that you drink liquor, do as such with some restraint. On the off chance that you drink, restrict your liquor utilization to close to two beverages for each day for men and one beverage for every day for ladies. One beverage rises to a 12-ounce lager, a 4-ounce glass of wine, 1.5 ounces of 80-proof alcohol, or 1 ounce of hard alcohol (100-proof). In the event that you drink in overabundance, get some answers concerning controlling liquor admission.

Drinking a lot of liquor can expand your blood pressure.

There is some association between blood pressure and these variables yet science has not demonstrated that they really cause hypertension.

STRESS

Being in an upsetting circumstance can incidentally expand your blood pressure, yet science has not demonstrated that push causes hypertension. A few researchers have noticed a relationship between coronary illness hazard and push in a man's life, wellbeing practices and financial status. How you manage anxiety may influence other, built up danger components for hypertension or coronary illness. Case in point, individuals under anxiety may gorge or eat a less solid eating routine, put off physical action, drink, smoke or abuse drugs. Discover approaches to diminish stress.

SMOKING AND SECOND-HAND SMOKE

Smoking briefly raises blood pressure and expands your danger of harmed arteries. The utilization of tobacco can be wrecking to your wellbeing, particularly in case you're as of now at danger for hypertension. Used smoke - introduction to other individuals' smoke - builds the danger of coronary illness for nonsmokers. Figure out how to kick the propensity.

REST APNEA

Around 12 million Americans have rest apnea, as per National Heart, Lung, and Blood Establishment gauges. Rest Apnea is a conceivably life-debilitating rest issue in which tissues in the throat crumple and hinder the aviation route. The mind compels the sleeper sufficiently conscious to hack or swallow air and open the trachea up once more. Be that as it may, then, the entire cycle starts from the very beginning once more. Stops in breathing can add to extreme weariness amid the day, build your dangers, and make it hard to perform errands that oblige sharpness. Rest apnea is additionally a danger element for such therapeutic issues right now pressure, heart failure, diabetes and stroke. Take in more about rest apnea.

In 5-10 percent of hypertension cases, the HBP is brought on by a prior issue. This sort of HBP is called auxiliary hypertension in light of the fact that another issue was available first.

Components that may prompt optional hypertension include:

- Kidney variation from the norm, including a tumor on the adrenal organ which is situated on top of the kidneys

- An auxiliary irregularity of the aorta (the vast blood vessel leaving the heart) that has existed since conception

- Narrowing of specific arteries

The uplifting news is that these prior issues can ordinarily be settled. Case in point, specialists can repair a contracted course that supplies blood to a kidney. When the main driver of optional hypertension is adjusted, blood pressure normally comes back to typical. For those with HBP, a physical exam and a few tests can help your specialist figure out if your hypertension is essential or optional hypertension. Hypertension is only one condition that expands your danger of coronary illness and stroke.

In upwards of 95% of reported hypertension cases in the U.S., the basic reason can't be resolved. This kind of hypertension is called "fundamental hypertension."

Despite the fact that key hypertension remains fairly baffling, it has been connected to certain danger elements. Hypertension has a tendency to keep running in families and is more inclined to influence men than ladies. Age and race additionally assume a part. In the United States, blacks are twice at this very moment whites to have hypertension, despite the fact that the whole starts to limit around age 44. After age 65, dark ladies have the most noteworthy occurrence of hypertension.

Hypertension can likewise be activated by tumors or different irregularities that cause the adrenal organs (little organs that sit on the kidneys) to discharge abundance measures of the hormones that lift blood pressure.

Contraception pills - particularly those containing estrogen - and pregnancy can help blood pressure that tightens blood vessels.

HOW IS BLOOD PRESSURE MEASURED?

To discover your blood pressure, two estimations are recorded amid a solitary pulse:

1. The level of pressure when your heart pumps blood through your arteries and around your body (systolic pressure): this is the point at which the pressure is most noteworthy, and

2. The level of pressure when your heart is resting before it pumps once more (diastolic pressure): this is the point at which the pressure is lea

Blood pressure is measured in millimeters of mercury (mmHg). The readings are given at this very moment or levels. The systolic perusing is initially, trailed by the diastolic perusing. For instance, if you're systolic perusing is 120mmHg and your diastolic perusing is 80mmHg, your blood pressure is 120 more than 80. This is generally composed presently.

WHAT ARE THE SIDE EFFECTS OF HYPERTENSION?

Typically, there are no particular manifestations which demonstrate that somebody has hypertension. Be that as it may, some populace reviews have demonstrated that a wide mixed bag of normal side effects, for example, rest unsettling influence, enthusiastic miracles, and dry mouth, are marginally plebian in individuals with higher pressures. The distinctions are little, notwithstanding. Going red in the face, or feeling flushed, is not demonstrative of hypertension.

MIGRAINE AND HYPERTENSION

On the off chance that you asked a hundred individuals what is the commonest side effect of hypertension; the chances are that the greater part would say cerebral pain. Indeed, not just do a great many people with hypertension not have migraines any more than whatever remains of us, yet when they do; it's normally not from the blood pressure. Just having an abnormal state of blood pressure inside your head does not typically deliver any side effects; in the event that you lift an overwhelming weight, your pressure may go up by 30 or 40 mm Hg, yet you don't get a cerebral pain.

What can bring about cerebral pain is muscle strain. Any muscle that is tensed for quite some time begins to hurt, and incessant pressure in the scalp or neck muscles is an extremely regular reason for cerebral pain. A study directed numerous years back shed some extremely intriguing light on the relationship in the middle of migraine and hypertension. Out of 104 individuals who had hypertension however were unconscious of it, just three volunteered that they had migraines, albeit another 14 let it be known when inquired. In any case, of 96 individuals who had been informed that they had hypertension, 71 said they had cerebral pains. The easiest clarification for this finding is that being informed that you have hypertension makes you begin to stress, and that this thusly causes the migraines.

There are a much littler number of patients, for the most part with high pressures, in whom cerebral pains are straightforwardly identified with the tallness of the blood pressure. In such people treating the blood pressure will diminish the side effects.

You can have HBP for a considerable length of time without knowing it. Amid this time, the condition can harm your heart, blood vessels, kidneys, and different parts of your body.

A few individuals just discover that they have HBP after the harm has brought about issues, for example, coronary illness, stroke, or kidney failure.

Knowing your blood pressure numbers is imperative, notwithstanding when you're feeling fine. On the off chance that your blood pressure is ordinary, you can work with your social insurance group to keep it that way. In the event that your blood pressure is too high, you can make moves to lower it. Bringing down your blood pressure will help diminish your danger for related wellbeing issues.

Chapter 2: High Blood Pressure – Dangers, Treatment & Prevention

THE RISKS BROUGHT ON BY HYPERTENSION

DEMENTIA

WHAT CAUSES IT?

Uncontrolled hypertension can bring about issues by harming and narrowing the blood vessels in your cerebrum. After some time, this raises the danger of a blood vessel getting to be blocked or blasting.

On the off chance that a blood can't convey vitality and oxygen to a piece of the cerebrum because of a blocked or burst blood vessel, a few cells in the mind may be harmed or even pass on.

This harm can once in a while influence a man's memory, considering, or dialect abilities. This is called vascular dementia.

BY WHAT MEANS WOULD YOU BE ABLE TO ANTICIPATE IT?

Receiving a sound way of life will help to moderate the development of harm to your blood vessels and will decrease your danger of creating vascular dementia. Likewise, on the off chance that you have a condition that may harm your blood vessels, (for example, diabetes, elevated cholesterol and heart issues) it is imperative to get them under control.

Having hypertension is a danger component for vascular dementia. On the off chance that you can bring down your blood pressure through way of life changes and drugs, you can diminish your danger.

Vascular dementia is most ordinarily brought on by the impacts of a stroke. You can bring down your danger of a stroke by keeping your blood pressure and cholesterol levels down.

In the event that you smoke, in the event that you have an unfortunate eating regimen, or on the off chance that you are overweight or not extremely dynamic, you ought to consider changing to a more solid way of life. This will help bring down your blood pressure, and bring down your danger of creating dementia.

STROKES

WHAT CAUSES IT?

Hypertension is a noteworthy reason for strokes in the UK. By bringing down your blood pressure, you can decrease your danger of building up a stroke. Uncontrolled hypertension can bring about issues by harming and narrowing the blood vessels in your cerebrum. After some time, this raises the danger of a blood vessel getting to be blocked or blasting.

On the off chance that blood can't convey vitality and oxygen to a piece of the mind because of a blocked or burst blood vessel, a few cells in the cerebrum may be harmed or even pass on. This is known as a stroke, and it can prompt inability and even passing.

By what method would you be able to avoid it?

Having hypertension is a noteworthy danger variable for stroke. On the off chance that you can bring down your blood pressure through way of life changes and drugs, you can lessen your danger.

DIABETES

WHAT CAUSES IT?

Around 25% of individuals with Sort 1 diabetes and 80% of individuals with Sort 2 diabetes have hypertension.

Having diabetes raises your danger of coronary illness, stroke, kidney infection and other wellbeing issues. Having hypertension likewise raises this danger. In the event that you have diabetes and hypertension together, this raises your danger of wellbeing issues much more

In the event that you have diabetes, your specialist will need to make certain that your blood pressure is extremely very much controlled. This implies that they will likely need your blood pressure to be beneath 130 more than 80

Individuals with diabetes and hypertension are here and there given the blood pressure meds known presently or Angiotensin receptor blockers, on the grounds that they are thought to help ensure the kidneys. Nonetheless, other blood pressure solutions can likewise be utilized.

By what means would you be able to anticipate it?

Numerous elements focus your danger of creating diabetes - your age, your ethnicity, or any family history of diabetes, for instance. Some of these things you can't take care of.

Be that as it may, you can help to bring down your danger of diabetes by taking after a solid way of life - for instance, by halting smoking, by eating a sound eating routine and keeping to a solid weight, and by getting more dynamic.

WEAK ARTERIES

WHAT CAUSES IT?

Hypertension can influence the capacity of the veins to open and close. On the off chance that your blood pressure is too high, the muscles in the supply route divider will react by pushing back harder. This will make them become greater, which makes your course dividers thicker.

Thicker arteries imply that there is less space for the blood to move through. This will raise your blood pressure significantly facilitate.

The higher your blood pressure is, the more noteworthy the chance that the additional pressure could make a frail artery burst. Likewise, the smaller your arteries are, the more prominent the danger that they could get to be blocked.

In the event that a course blasts or gets to be obstructed, the a piece of the body that gets its blood from that supply route will be famished of the vitality and oxygen it needs and the cells in the influenced region will bite the dust.

On the off chance that the burst artery supplies the brain then the outcome is a stroke. In the event that the burst supply route supplies a piece of the heart, then that region of heart muscle will bite the dust, creating a heart assault.

BY WHAT MEANS WOULD YOU BE ABLE TO COUNTERACT IT?

You can help your veins to stay solid by keeping your blood pressure controlled and by taking after a sound way of life.

Adhering to a good diet will give your body the vitality and supplements it needs to keep it in great condition. Getting dynamic will likewise keep your heart and blood vessels fit and solid.

A large portion of the prescriptions used to treat hypertension work to keep the arteries more extensive. They do this by following up on specifically on the muscles in the conduit divider, or by controlling hormones that follow up on these muscles.

HEART FAILURE

WHAT CAUSES IT?

In the event that you have hypertension, this implies that your heart needs to work harder to push blood round your body. To adapt to this additional exertion, your heart gets to be thicker and stiffer, which makes it less ready to carry out its occupation.

In the event that your heart is not ready to pump and in addition it ought to, this is called heart failure. Heart failure can bring about additional liquid to develop in the body, and can likewise bring about a sporadic pulse. It doesn't imply that your heart is going to quit working; however it is a genuine condition.

In what capacity would you be able to avert it?

Heart failure can't be cured, yet there are medicines accessible. It is imperative to discover the reason for heart failure so that your specialist is not simply treating the indications.

Some blood pressure meds can help treat heart failure, for instance diuretics can help to decrease liquid develop. Pro inhibitors and Angiotensin receptor blockers can likewise offer assistance.

Certain meds called beta-blockers are regularly utilized, yet these are generally not the same as the sorts that are utilized to treat hypertension. Different pharmaceuticals can likewise be utilized.

You can help enhance the strength of your heart by rolling out way of life improvements - ceasing smoking, eliminating liquor, or being more dynamic (it doesn't should be excessively vigorous; strolling consistently will help your heart).

EXPANDED HEART

WHAT CAUSES IT?

In the event that you have hypertension, this implies that your heart needs to work harder to push blood round your body. To adapt to this additional exertion, your heart muscles get to be thicker and stiffer, which can make the heart get to be broadened.

An amplified heart won't pump and additionally it ought to, and this can bring about you issues. Specifically, a broadened heart is a typical reason for heart failure.

In what manner would you be able to anticipate it?

An amplified heart can be dealt with and, for a few individuals; it is conceivable to diminish the broadened region after some time.

A significant number of the prescriptions used to treat hypertension will likewise decrease heart muscle size on the off chance that it is expanded. Specifically, Expert inhibitors and Angiotensin receptor blockers can be extremely powerful.

KIDNEY DISEASE

WHAT CAUSES IT?

How sound your kidneys are can influence your blood pressure, and the other way around. This implies that in the event that you have hypertension, then you are more prone to have kidney infection. Moreover, in the event that you have kidney illness, this can once in a while cause hypertension.

The greatest wellbeing danger for individuals with kidney ailment is not really kidney failure. Individuals with kidney malady are considerably more liable to create coronary illness or have a stroke. So in the event that you have kidney infection you have to keep your heart and blood vessels sound. Controlling your blood pressure is a vital approach to do this.

By what method would you be able to avert it?

Your specialist will have the capacity to exhort you about rolling out way of life improvements to help diminish the impacts of kidney ailment. They may propose any of the accompanying:

- eating a healthier eating routine, and decreasing the measure of salt you eat

- increasing the measure of normal activity you get

- stopping smoking

- losing weight in the event that you have to

- Cutting back on liquor.

And helping your kidneys, this way of life changes will help bring down your blood pressure and keep your blood sugar controlled. This will likewise help to decrease your danger of coronary illness and stroke.

On the off chance that your kidney malady is more extreme your specialist may recommend an uncommon eating routine to lessen the measure of waste items your body produces. This will give your kidneys less work to do.

In the event that you have kidney sickness, it is essential that you don't utilize salt substitutes, for example, Lo-Salt. These items contain a ton of potassium and, if your kidneys are not living up to expectations appropriately, potassium can develop, which can prompt wellbeing issues.

PERIPHERAL ARTERY DISEASE

WHAT CAUSES IT?

In the event that hypertension is left untreated for quite a while, it can put additional strain on the arteries in your arms and legs and may bring about the blood vessels in the legs to thin, bringing on excruciating spasms.

Hypertension can bring about your arteries to wind up more restricted. They can likewise harm the veins, and greasy stores can develop around the regions of harm. These stores make the arteries smaller still and these outcomes in poor course in the legs and feet. These issues are known right now ailment (Cushion)

In what capacity would you be able to counteract it?

It is conceivable to back off the movement of fringe artery ailment (Cushion) and once in a while reverse it rolling out positive improvements to your way of life.

Customary strolling for 30 minutes a day can offer assistance. In the event that this is a lot for you to do at the same time, you may be requested that development the time you can stroll for before you feel torment. As it were, stroll until you feel agony, rest for a couple of minutes and after that keep on strolling until you have to rest once more, until you have strolled for 30 minutes.

Eating less immersed fats and trans-fats (which develop in the conduits) and supplanting them with unsaturated fats will help divert the greasy stores from the arteries. On the off chance that you are overweight, shedding pounds will offer assistance. Surrendering smoking will likewise help enormously.

SWOLLEN ANKLES

WHAT CAUSES IT?

Hypertension makes your heart specialist harder than it expected to sometime recently. Over the space of numerous years, this additional exertion can prompt the heart muscle getting to be thicker and less powerful at pushing the blood round. This permits liquid to develop in your lower legs and ankles, which make them, swell up.

Swollen lower legs can likewise be a symptom of some blood pressure meds, specifically calcium channel blockers. These prescriptions make your little blood vessels open more extensive and, in a few individuals, this can bring about more liquid to hole out of the blood vessels into the tissues. This liquid will gather around your lower legs.

In what manner would you be able to forestall it?

Diuretic pharmaceuticals build the measure of liquid evacuated by your kidneys and this can help to dispose of any overabundance liquid from the body. This uproots the development of liquid from the tissues in your lower legs.

In the event that your lower leg swelling is because of taking calcium channel blockers, decreasing the dosage of your medication will typically offer assistance. On the other hand, if your blood pressure is not completely controlled, your specialist may endorse you a diuretic to help bring down your blood pressure further and evacuate the overabundance liquid.

You can help to diminish the swelling by sitting with your legs lifted up. This lets your blood stream all the more unreservedly and ought to help lessen the swelling.

ERECTILE DYSFUNCTION

WHAT CAUSES IT?

Erectile dysfunction is all the more regularly known right now. It is the failure to get an erection sufficiently enduring, or sufficiently firm, for penetrative sex.

Men with hypertension can at times experience erectile dysfunction however, for large portions of them; it can be dealt with adequately.

A typical reason for erectile dysfunction (barrenness) is harm to the coating of the arteries to the penis, so they neglect to open up and let the blood into reinforce an erection.

Blood pressure can harm your arteries by making them get to be thicker, or even to blast. This can limit blood stream to your penis, which might then bring about erectile dysfunction.

Some blood pressure prescriptions can likewise bring about erectile dysfunction. Thiaziden diuretics and beta-blockers are well on the way to bring about issues, yet this is not a typical impact of these medications and won't happen to everybody. In the event that you are taking both of these meds and are stressed over erectile dysfunction, your GP may have the capacity to change your prescriptions.

By what method would you be able to avoid it?

On the off chance that erectile dysfunction (weakness) is brought on by hypertension, then bringing down blood pressure through pharmaceuticals and way of life changes ought to treat the issue successfully.

On the off chance that the issue is brought about by blood pressure pharmaceuticals, your specialist may have the capacity to change your dosage or change you to an alternate pharmaceutical. Try not to quit taking your meds without addressing your specialist first.

In the event that issues with erectile dysfunction proceed, there are medications accessible to manage it specifically. Identify with your specialist about what alternatives may be a good fit for you.

PREGNANCY AND HYPERTENSION

In the event that you grow hypertension amid your pregnancy, your blood pressure ought to come back to its ordinary level after your child is conceived. Blood pressure levels can likewise rise strongly taking after the conveyance of a child, and this can proceed for a couple of weeks. It is critical to screen your blood pressure firmly after you have conceived an offspring, to verify that it comes back to typical.

Hypertension in a past pregnancy does not imply that you will have it again in a later pregnancy, yet you will have a somewhat higher shot of creating it than other ladies.

In the event that you as of now have hypertension and you get to be pregnant, or in the event that you want to have a child, it is imperative to converse with your specialist. It is conceivable to have a fruitful and solid pregnancy, however in the event that you do have hypertension you have a somewhat more prominent shot of entanglements than other ladies. So you should be checked more nearly than ladies who don't have hypertension.

Likewise, your specialist may wish you to change your blood pressure solutions, or even request that you quit taking them amid your pregnancy. It is felt that some blood pressure meds, for example, Expert inhibitors and Angiotensin receptor blockers may confine an infant's development.

PREGNANCY AND MENOPAUSE

Hormone substitution treatment (HRT) medications incorporate the hormone estrogen. Estrogens can bring about an ascent in blood pressure, which is the reason a few types of the prophylactic pill can raise blood pressure. In any case, there's still some open deliberation about whether there's a connection in the middle of HRT and an ascent in blood pressure.

Late research has demonstrated that more established ladies who were taking HRT (hormone substitution treatment) and who likewise had coronary illness or had a stroke were marginally more prone to have further heart issues than ladies who were not taking HRT.

In the event that you have coronary illness or have had a stroke, then taking HRT would not be prompted, unless you are experiencing extremely serious indications. On the off chance that this is the situation, then HRT ought to just be brought after dialog with a master.

On the off chance that you do choose to take HRT, then it is imperative that you attempt to keep up a sound way of life, at this very moment lessen your general danger of stroke or heart assault. This implies not smoking; being the right weight for your stature, eating a low-salt, low-fat eating regimen with bunches of products of the soil and being dynamic.

On the off chance that you have hypertension and you are taking HRT (hormone substitution treatment) you ought to have your blood pressure checked like clockwork.

On the off chance that you don't have hypertension and are taking HRT, you ought to likewise have your blood pressure checked consistently presently ascend amid the menopause at this very moment more than when you get older.

CHAPTER 3: BLOOD PRESSURE – CONTROLLING IT THE NATURAL WAY

THE ROLE OF DIET

NOURISHMENTS THAT BRING DOWN YOUR BLOOD PRESSURE

Ever consider how to lower blood pressure actually? Sodium has dependably been the blood pressure bogeyman—shakes the greater part of it from your eating regimen and you'll be safe. However, examine now demonstrates that its generally presently pick sustenance normally low in sodium and high in no less than two of the three force minerals: calcium, magnesium, and potassium. Include these very much adjusted nourishments to your eating regimen to cut your danger of stroke and heart assault about down the middle.

WHITE BEANS

One measure of white beans gives 13% of the calcium, 30% of the magnesium, and 24% of the potassium you require consistently.

You can utilize this solace nourishment in side dishes, soups, and entrées. At this very moment wellspring of protein, it's an extraordinary decision for vegans. Pick no-salt included or very much flushed low-sodium canned white beans, or cook dried beans overnight in a moderate cooker.

PORK TENDERLOIN

Three ounces of pork tenderloin give 6% of the magnesium and 15% of the potassium you require consistently.

Meat sweethearts, celebrate! This incline cut gives a lot of substantial flavor and fulfillment without the over-burden of immersed fat found in fattier sorts of meat and pork. Cook bigger tenderloins (or do a few on the barbecue or in the broiler) and store scraps in the icebox or cooler for quick weeknight suppers.

RECIPE

Basic Meal Pork Loin

PREP TIME: 5 minutes

Aggregate TIME: 60 minutes, 30 minutes

SERVINGS: 4 (with scraps)

- 1 vast pork loin, trimmed (around 10 lbs)

- 8 cloves garlic

- ¼ cups olive oil

- Salt and naturally ground pepper to taste

Preheat the broiler to 350°F. Rub the pork with garlic and olive oil. Season with salt and pepper for taste. Coat a 9" x 13" heating dish with cooking shower. Place the pork in the readied heating dish. Heat for more or less 60 minutes, or until a thermometer embedded in the middle registers 145°F. Expel the pork from the broiler and let it remain for 15 minutes prior to cutting. Cut it into 8 cuts; wrap the rest firmly in plastic wrap and store in the fridge. Serve with pureed potatoes and a green serving of mixed greens.

Nutrients (per serving) 230 cal, 23 g professional, 0 g carb, 0 g fiber, 12 g fat, 5 g sat fat, 53 mg sodium

SANS FAT PLAIN YOGURT

One measure of sans fat plain yogurt gives 49% of the calcium, 12% of the magnesium, and 18% of the potassium you require consistently.

Cool and velvety, yogurt is a star fixing in mineral-rich breakfasts, in sauces and serving of mixed greens dressings, and even in entrées. Most brands of customary yogurt have a tendency to be somewhat higher in calcium than Greek assortments.

KIWIFRUIT

One kiwifruit gives 2% of the calcium, 7% of the magnesium, and 9% of the potassium you require consistently.

Kiwifruit is accessible year-round in markets, hailing from California plantations November through May and from New Zealand June through October. (Kiwifruit was named after New Zealand's local kiwi winged creature, whose cocoa, fluffy coat looks like the skin of this natural product.) Ready kiwis can be put away in the refrigerator or on your counter. They contain more vitamin C than a same-size serving of orange cuts.

PEACHES AND NECTARINES

One medium peach or nectarine gives 1% of the calcium, 3% of the magnesium, and 8% of the potassium you require consistently.

Solidified unsweetened peach cuts are an incredible distinct option for crisp peaches and nectarines. Simply defrost early or, for smoothies, essentially hurl in the blender.

BANANAS

One medium banana gives 1% of the calcium, 8% of the magnesium, and 12% of the potassium you require consistently.

No compelling reason to hurl delicate bananas when the skin turns chestnut. Peel, pack, and stop for utilization in smoothies. (Extra: bananas help lower anxiety hormones in the blood

KALE

One measure of kale, crude or cooked, gives 9% of the calcium, 6% of the magnesium, and 9% of the potassium you require consistently.

Low in calories, kale is generally viewed as a super food on the grounds that it contains a major dosage of cell-securing cancer prevention agents and alpha-Linolenic corrosive, a plant-based great fat that cools irritation. Slender, fragile infant kale leaves are an awesome option for plates of mixed greens.

RED BELL PEPPER

One measure of crude red bell pepper gives 1% of the calcium, 4% of the magnesium, and 9% of the potassium you require consistently.

Red bell peppers keep in the fridge for up to 10 days. Store wrapped in a marginally sodden paper towel so they don't dry out. You can solidify additional items to utilize later in cooked dishes.

BROCCOLI

One measure of cooked broccoli gives 6% of the calcium, 8% of the magnesium, and 14% of the potassium you require consistently.

This cruciferous veggie is likewise an acclaimed wellspring of disease battling phytonutrient called glucosinolates. You can substitute solidified broccoli in numerous cooked entrées and side dishes.

Recipe

BROCCOLI-SHELLED SALAD

SERVINGS: 4

- ¼ c white wine vinegar

- 3 Tbsp canola oil

- 3 Tbsp nutty spread

- 1 Tbsp decreased sodium soy sauce

- ½ tsp salt

- 1 lb broccoli, tops cut into little florets and stems peeled and hacked

- ¼ c dried fruits, cranberries, or raisins

- ¼ c broiled peanuts, hacked

Whisk together vinegar, oil, nutty spread, soy sauce, and salt in an extensive dish. Hurl with broccoli and dried products of the soil with salt to taste. Serve finished with peanuts. It can be made up to 2 days ahead.

Nutrients (per serving) 280 cal, 9 g expert, 17 g carb, 7 g fiber, 5 g sugars, 21 g fat, 2.5 g sat fat, 510 mg sodium

QUINOA

A half-measure of cooked quinoa gives 1.5% of the calcium, 15% of the magnesium, and 4.5% of the potassium you require consistently.

There's a reason the United Countries proclaimed 2013 the Universal Year of Quinoa. This high-protein entire grain has a mellow yet nutty flavor, contains a mixture of wellbeing securing phytonutrient alongside a great measure of magnesium, and cooks in under a fraction of the time it takes to make cocoa rice. Quinoa is without gluten, making it an extraordinary choice in case you're gluten bigoted or have celiac sickness. The most broadly accessible quinoa is a brilliant beige shading, however red and dark assortments are additionally accessible and worth an attempt.

Recipe

Best Fundamental Quinoa

PREP TIME: 15 minutes

Aggregate TIME: 40 minutes

SERVINGS: 4 (with remains)

- ½ c additional virgin olive oil

- 3 c hacked green Chime pepper

- 3 c hacked yellow onion

- 3 c hacked celery

- 1 tsp salt

- 6 c quinoa

- 12 c decreased sodium without fat chicken juices

- 12 scallions, cut daintily

Heat the olive oil in an additional extensive soup pot. Include the Chime pepper, onion, celery, and salt. Cook, mixing oftentimes, for 4 minutes, or until the pepper begins to relax. Include the quinoa. Blend to coat. Include the soup. Heat to the point of boiling and spread, and then decrease the warmth to low. Stew for 20 minutes, or until all the fluid is retained. Off warmth, blend in the scallions.

Nutrition (per serving) 249 cal, 7 g ace, 37 g carb, 4 g fiber, 8 g fat, 1 g sat fat, 566 mg sodium

AVOCADO

One-a large portion of an avocado gives 1% of the calcium, 5% of the magnesium, and 10% of the potassium you require consistently.

Notwithstanding pressure-mitigating minerals and heart-sound monounsaturated fats, avocados contain wellbeing advancing carotenoids. Peel painstakingly; the dim green tissue simply under an avocado's weak skin contains a lot of these illness battling mixes.

Recipe
SERVINGS: 4

- 4 slight cuts red onion, isolated into rings

- 2 oranges

- 2 avocados

- 3 Tbsp olive oil

- 2 Tbsp cleaved crisp mint

- 1 Tbsp crisply crushed lemon juice (about ½ sm lemon)

- ¼ tsp salt

Absorb onion little bowl of ice water to fresh. Peel oranges with blade, evacuating all of white essence. Cut across into dainty wheels. Pit, peel, and cut avocados and put in medium dish. Channel onion well and add to bowl alongside oranges, olive oil, mint, lemon squeeze, and salt. Hurl to coat.

Nutrition (per serving) 286 cal, 3 g master, 18 g carb, 9 g fiber, 25 g fat, 3.5 g sat fat, 0 mg chol, 135 mg sodium

Dietary changes to naturally bring down your BP without medications

Decrease exorbitant starch admission, particularly refined carbs and sugars.

A standout amongst the most noteworthy patrons to high blood pressure is high blood sugar and insulin resistance. Some proof proposes that neurotic changes in glucose and insulin digestion system fundamentally influence the improvement and clinical course of hypertension, and consequently ought to be essential focuses for dietary mediation. Chronically high blood sugar, hyperinsulinemia, and high triglycerides are significantly more normal in people with hypertension than those with typical blood pressure, and one of the significant benefactors to every one of the three of these conditions is an abundance admission of carb, especially refined grains and sugars.

Moreover, abundance admission of sugar-sweetened refreshments like pop, sweet tea, and other sugary beverages has been demonstrated to specifically impact blood pressure. Removing these refreshments ought to be the initial phase in any hypertension treatment, and can likewise help with shedding abundance weight and diminishing high blood sugar – both issues that further add to hypertension. Also, don't think changing to Eating regimen will help either, since falsely sweetened drinks likewise add to hypertension.

Make certain to modify your starch admission to your needs and wellbeing objectives, and get your sugars from supplement thick entire sustenance like products of the soil vegetables.

Expand admission of helpful minerals like potassium, magnesium, and calcium.

While most customary medicinal experts will prescribe sodium limitation at this very moment strategy for blood pressure diminishment, it creates the impression that concentrating on eating nourishments rich in different macro minerals is more painful than entirely concentrating on staying away from sodium. More imperative than general sodium admission is the sodium-to-potassium proportion; subsequently, eating a high-potassium eating regimen is a superior technique than eating a low-sodium diet.

Those with hypertension ought to expect to get no less than 4,700 milligrams of potassium for each day. In the event that you have hypertension and are uncertain about the sufficiency of your potassium admission, utilize a sustenance journal for 3 days and break down your normal potassium consumption.

Likewise, don't go too low carb when diminishing your starch consumption – a hefty portion of the best wellsprings of potassium and magnesium are bland vegetables like white and sweet potatoes, or natural products like plantains and bananas. White potatoes are particularly great wellsprings of blood pressure-bringing down minerals like potassium and magnesium; theoretically you could eat three huge heated potatoes every day to effectively meet your potassium needs while just devouring around 180 grams of sugar.

Eat grass-bolstered dairy items like ghee, spread, and cheddar.
Past being a decent wellspring of calcium, full-fat grass-nourished dairy has another commitment to the treatment of hypertension: vitamin K2. While this supplement is not really examined by traditional restorative experts, preparatory information recommends K2 may be a standout amongst the most imperative supplements to incorporate in an ailment avoiding eating regimen. Vitamin K2 may be defensive against osteoporosis, cardiovascular sickness, malignancy, and the sky is the limit from there, so it's certainly a supplement you ought to be hoping to get enough of regardless of what your wellbeing circumstance.

Vitamin K2 might likewise be defensive against hypertension. While there haven't yet been any studies straightforwardly measuring K2's impacts on blood pressure rationale would recommend that this supplement could help anticipate high blood pressure by diminishing vascular solidness and blood vessel calcification.

EAT NO LESS THAN ONE POUND OF GREASY FISH EVERY WEEK.

Greasy fish is high in key omega-3 fats, and these fats have been indicated to lessen the danger of hypertension and cardiovascular occasions in numerous studies. A meta-examination showed that fish oil supplementation might essentially decrease both systolic and diastolic blood pressure. On the other hand, taking fish oil supplements to get your omega-3 fats is not a perfect technique, since a few studies recommend that high measurements of fish oil may expand cardiovascular and all out mortality, particularly when utilized for over four years.

DRINK TEA.

Routine tea drinking may help lessen blood pressure, presently examine generally led in areas where tea is a critical segment of the day by day diet. There are a few teas that may be more powerful at decreasing blood pressure than others, nonetheless, and jazzed tea may bring blood pressure up in the short term. (On the off chance that you are taking physician endorsed drugs, converse with your medicinal services supplier before drinking these natural teas.)

HIBISCUS TEA has been exhibited to lessen blood pressure in pre-and gently hypertensive grown-ups. Hibiscus is a little tree with red blooms that are rich in flavonoids, minerals, and different supplements.

Recipe

- 2 quarts water

- 3/4 to 1 glass sugar (contingent upon how sweet you would like it to be)

- 1 glass dried hibiscus blooms

- 1/2 cinnamon stick (discretionary)

- A couple flimsy cuts ginger (discretionary)

- Allspice berries (discretionary)

- Lime juice (discretionary)

• Orange or lime cuts for enhancement

Technique

Put some the water and the sugar in a medium pot. Include cinnamon, ginger cuts, and/or a couple allspice berries on the off chance that you would like. Heat until bubbling and the sugar has disintegrated. Expel from warmth. Blend in the dried hibiscus blossoms. Spread and let sit for 20 minutes. Strain into a pitcher and toss the utilized hibiscus blooms, ginger, cinnamon, and/or allspice berries. Include remaining some water (or on the off chance that you need to cool the beverage rapidly, ice and water) to the concentrate, and chill. Then again you can include ice and chilled pop water for a bubbly form. Include a little lime juice for a more punch-like flavor.

Serve over ice with a cut of orange or lime.

Hawthorn tea might likewise be compelling at this very moment pressure-lessening refreshment, and the plant has been utilized to regard coronary illness as far back right now century. The cell reinforcement rich tea may help enlarge blood vessels and enhance blood stream. Dosing rules have not been built up, but rather three containers a day is suggested by some wellbeing experts.

Gotu kola tea may be another useful tea in bringing down blood pressure, particularly on account of venous inadequacy. It is accepted that Gotu kola may help with the upkeep of connective tissue, which reinforces debilitated veins and aides enhance dissemination. Once more, three mugs every day is the present suggestion for this tea.

At long last, oolong and green tea may be advantageous for bringing down high blood pressure.

EAT MORE BEETS.

A few specialists theorize that a noteworthy reason the DASH eating routine is gainful for bringing down blood pressure is that the substance of inorganic nitrate in specific vegetables and natural products gives a physiologic substrate to diminishment to nitrite, nitric oxide, and other metabolic items that deliver vasodilatation, abatement blood pressure, and bolster cardiovascular capacity.

DASH DIET

DASH remains for Dietary Ways to deal with Stop Hypertension. The DASH eating routine is a deep rooted way to deal with good dieting that is intended to help treat or counteract high blood pressure (hypertension).

You can pick the form of the eating routine that meets your wellbeing needs:

- Standard DASH diet. You can devour up to 2,300 milligrams (mg) of sodium a day.

- Lower sodium DASH diet. You can devour up to 1,500 mg of sodium a day.

Both variants of the DASH eating routine intend to diminish the measure of sodium in your eating routine contrasted and what you may get in a more customary eating routine, which can sum to an astounding 3,500 mg of sodium a day or more.

GRAINS: 6 TO 8 SERVINGS A DAY

Grains incorporate bread, cereal, rice and pasta. Illustrations of one serving of grains incorporate 1 cut entire wheat bread, 1 ounce (oz.) dry grain, or 1/2 container cooked oat, rice or pasta.

VEGETABLES: 4 TO 5 SERVINGS A DAY

Tomatoes, carrots, broccoli, sweet potatoes, greens and different vegetables are brimming with fiber, vitamins, and such minerals right now magnesium. Cases of one serving incorporate 1 container crude verdant green vegetables or 1/2 glass cut-up crude or cooked vegetables.

NATURAL PRODUCTS: 4 TO 5 SERVINGS A DAY

Numerous natural products require little arrangement to turn into a sound piece of a feast or nibble. Like vegetables, they're stuffed with fiber, potassium and magnesium and are regularly low in fat — special cases incorporate avocados and coconuts. Samples of one serving incorporate 1 medium natural product or 1/2 container crisp, solidified or canned organic product or 4 ounces of juice.

DAIRY: 2 TO 3 SERVINGS A DAY

Milk, yogurt, cheddar and other dairy items are real wellsprings of calcium, vitamin D and protein. Yet, the key is to verify that you pick dairy items that are low fat or sans fat on the grounds that else they can be a noteworthy wellspring of fat — and a large portion of it is immersed. Illustrations of one serving incorporate 1 glass skim or 1 percent drain, 1 container yogurt, or 1/2 oz. cheddar.

INCLINE MEAT, POULTRY AND FISH: 6 OR LESS SERVINGS A DAY

Meat can be a rich wellspring of protein, B vitamins, iron and zinc. But since even incline assortments contain fat and cholesterol, don't make them a pillar of your eating routine — decrease regular meat partitions by 33% or one-half and heap on the vegetables. Cases of one serving incorporate 1 oz. cooked skinless poultry, fish or incline meat or 1 egg.

PHYSICAL ACTION TO LOWER BLOOD PRESSURE AND SHED POUNDS

A strong collection of proof demonstrates that men and ladies of all age groups who are physically dynamic have a diminished danger of growing high blood pressure. Discoveries from various studies demonstrate that practice can lower blood pressure as much right now can. Individuals with mellow and modestly raised blood pressure who practices 30 to an hour three to four days for every week (strolling, running, cycling, or a blend) may have the capacity to essentially diminish their blood pressure readings.

GO FOR POWER STROLLS

Hypertensive patients who went for wellness strolls at a lively pace brought down blood pressure by very nearly 8 mm/hg more than 6 mm/hg. Activity helps the heart use oxygen all the more productively, so it doesn't act at this very moment pump blood. Get an incredible cardio workout of no less than 30 minutes on most days of the week. Take a stab at expanding speed or separation to give your heart a superior workout.

BLOOD PRESSURE, BREATHING, AND ANXIETY ADMINISTRATION

Blood pressure increments when a man is under enthusiastic anxiety and pressure, yet regardless of whether mental mediations went for anxiety decrease can decline blood pressure in patients with hypertension is not clear.

In any case, late studies recommend that antiquated unwinding strategies that incorporate controlled breathing and tender physical movement, for example, yoga, Qigong, and Kendo, are gainful. Individuals with gentle hypertension who honed these mending procedures day by day for a few months experienced noteworthy declines in their blood pressure, had lower levels of anxiety hormones, and were less on edge.

The aftereffects of a late little study propose that an everyday routine of moderate breathing (15 minutes a day for 8 weeks) realized a generous diminishment in blood pressure. Be that as it may, these discoveries should be affirmed in bigger and better-outlined studies before these antiquated recuperating procedures are prescribed at this very moment pharmacological ways to deal with treating hypertension. Still, conceivable advantages, combined with negligible dangers, make these tender practices a beneficial action to join into a sound way of life.

LITTLE CHANGES AND ACTIVITIES TO ADOPT TO BRING DOWN YOUR BLOOD PRESSURE

BE SALT KEEN

Certain gatherings of individuals—the elderly, African Americans, and those with a family history of high blood pressure—are more probable than others to have blood pressure that is especially salt (or sodium) delicate. But since there's no real way to tell whether any one individual is sodium delicate, everybody ought to bring down his sodium admission. How far? To 1,500 mg day by day, about a large portion of the normal American consumption. (A large portion of a teaspoon of salt contains around 1,200 mg of sodium.) Cutting sodium implies more than going simple on the saltshaker, which contributes only 15% of the sodium in the average American diet. Look for sodium in prepared nourishments. That is the place a large portion of the sodium in your eating regimen originates from, she says. Season your food with flavors, herbs, lemon, and without salt flavoring mixes.

ENJOY DIM CHOCOLATE

Dull chocolate mixed bags contain flavanols that make blood vessels more versatile. In one study, 18% of patients who ate it consistently saw blood pressure diminish. Have 1/2 ounces day by day (verify it contains no less than 70 percent cocoa).

DRINK (A BIT) LIQUOR

As per an audit of 15 studies, the less you drink, the bring down your blood pressure will drop—to a point. An investigation, found that light drinking (characterized as one-quarter to one-a large portion of a beverage for every day for a lady) might really lessen blood pressure more than no beverages every day. One "beverage" is 12 ounces of brew, 5 ounces of wine, or 1.5 ounces of spirits. Different studies have likewise found that direct drinking—up to one drink a day for a lady, two for a man—can lower dangers of coronary illness. High levels of liquor are obviously impeding. Be that as it may, direct liquor is defensive of the heart. In the event that you are going to drink, drink reasonably.

WORK (SOMEWHAT) LESS

Putting in over 41 hours for every week at the workplace raises your danger of hypertension by 15%, as indicated by an investigation of 24,205 California inhabitants. Additional time makes it difficult to practice and eat healthy. It might be hard to check out super at a very early stage in today's extreme financial times, yet attempt to leave at an average hour—so you can go to the rec center or cook a sound feast—right now conceivable. Set an end-of-day message on your PC as a suggestion to turn it off and go home.

Unwind With Music

Need to cut down your blood pressure some more than pharmaceutical or way of life changes can do alone? The right tunes can help, as indicated by analysts at the College of Florence in Italy. They asked 28 grown-ups who were at that point taking hypertension pills to listen to calming traditional, Celtic, or Indian music for 30 minutes every day while breathing gradually. Following a week, the audience members had brought down their normal systolic perusing by 3.2 focuses; after a month, readings were down 4.4 focuses.

Look for Help for Wheezing

Now is the ideal time to regard your accomplice's protestations and get that wheezing looked at? Noisy, ceaseless wheezes are one of the fundamental side effects of obstructive rest apnea (OSA). College of Alabama specialists found that numerous rest apnea sufferers likewise had high levels of aldosterone, a hormone that can help blood pressure. Truth be told, it's evaluated that a large portion out of every other person on earth with rest apnea have high blood pressure. On the off chance that you have rest apnea, you may encounter numerous brief yet possibly life-undermining interferences in your breathing while you rest. Notwithstanding uproarious wheezing, extreme daytime tiredness and early morning cerebral pains are likewise great intimations. In the event that you have high blood pressure, inquire as to whether OSA could be behind it; treating rest apnea may lower aldosterone levels and enhance BP.

Bounce for Soy

A study from Flow: Diary of the American Heart Affiliation found surprisingly that supplanting a percentage of the refined starches in your eating routine with sustenance high in soy or milk protein, for example, low-fat dairy, can cut down systolic blood pressure on the off chance that you have hypertension or pre-hypertension.

CONCLUSION

This book was made to provide you with all the information on blood pressure in one same place so that you won't have to look around in different places for recipes and techniques on how to measure your blood pressure or the dangers it brings about.

We have compiled this book for your knowledge and for your comfort and we hope that this book has provided you what you came looking for. We hope this book has enabled you to live a healthy and balanced life with a stable blood pressure that is well under your control.

We wish you the very best of luck for all your future endeavors and want to thank you for downloading this book!

Thank you!

www.ingramcontent.com/pod-product-compliance
Lightning Source LLC
Chambersburg PA
CBHW030506170726
47990CB00008BA/3073